# Lose Your Weight Naturally
# The Way I Lost: How I lost 10kgs or 22 pounds in 14 days

by Dinesh Kumar

<h1 style="text-align:center">Prologue:</h1>

This book describes the complete fact about how I lost 10 kgs weight in 14 days with the help of Hatha Yoga, Pranayama, Mindful Meditation, Proper Diet plan and Law of attraction.

I followed 14 days plan for losing weight.

Day 1

I woke up at 4 am.
I did Kapalbhati Pranayama for 5 minutes.
Then I did Anulom Vilom Pranayama for 5 minutes.
Then I did Bhastrika Pranayama for 5 minutes.

Then I had 1 litre warm water with juice of half lemon and 1 spoon honey.

Then I did Jal Neti.

Then 7 am I did Kunjal Kriya.

9 am I had breakfast. In my breakfast I had 2 multigrain bread or roti, Yogurt, 1 glass cabbage juice and Boiled Cabbage as a vegetable, and lots of Salad.
In my salad, I had fine chopped cabbage leaves, 2 tomatoes, 2 carrots, 1 radish, 1 apple, 2 onions, 2 cloves of garlic, half spoon honey, two almonds, two walnuts and 2 sesame seeds laddu made in Jaggery.

Afternoon, I had 200gms of boiled broccoli with pinch of rock salt, 200 gms of Papaya, 2 pear, 2 apple and 1 cloves, 2 almonds and 2 walnuts and two seasame seeds laddu made in Jaggery.

Night I had a glass of mushroom onion soup, 200 gms of boiled cabbage with a pinch of rock salt, 200 gms yogurt and 2 pear, 1 apple and 200 gms of chopped pineapple, 200gms papayas and 2 seasame seeds laddu made in Jaggery.

I consumed 7-8 litre solarised water daily.

When water kept in a coloured container is exposed to sunlight, it absorbs the vibrational energy of that particular colour. This process is called solarizing or energising water. To reap the benefits of the particular colour, this water can be drunk or used for bathing. An unexpected benefit of solarized water of a particular color is weight loss.

How to make solarized water
Things you will need: A plain glass, coloured filter, rubber band, mineral water/spring water and muslin/cotton fabric.

How to make: Attach the chosen colour filter to the glass with the help of a rubber band. Fill the glass with mineral water and cover the top with muslin/cotton cloth.
Place this glass in sunlight. Instead of a coloured filter, you can use coloured glass but in this case, the colour should be strong enough and should not be light in shade.
This depends on how strong the sun is, like in summer, the process may take only a couple of hours but in winter, it may take an entire day. Solarized water can be kept in the fridge for up to five hours. Oils can also be solarized in a similar way and can be used for a massage later.

Colour for weight loss
As different colours serve different purposes, the colour good for weight loss is yellow. You can use a yellow colour tumbler or use a yellow colour filter to solarize water with this colour. Yellow colour is considered as the weight corrective colour. You can have a glass of solarized yellow water half an hour before having your meals to aid weight loss. Not only weight loss, yellow colour

also helps to cleanse your skin, prevent urine infection, helps in concentration, increases alertness and works as a laxative.

As having a good digestive system is one of the first steps to lose weight, you can also use orange tumbler to solarize water in order to improve digestion, relieve menstrual pain, reduce cramps and lift depression.

I followed this routine for 14 days (except the Kunjal kriya that I did once in 3 days) and after 14 days  I lost 10 kgs with a shining bright face, flat tummy and glowing skin.

Losing weight is not a very difficult thing, if one regularly follows a routine, a proper diet chart; and does exercises. If you think that you need to lose weight, first, you have to change your food habits. For that, you need to follow a proper diet chart, which you should follow every day. Try to eat healthy food, such as green vegetables, fresh fruits, fruit juices, cereals, oats, skimmed milk, etc. Avoid sugar, oily and spicy foods, junk food, and other high-calorie diet, as these give rise to obesity, and are not good for health.

Overweight has major health issues, including type 2 diabetes, sleep apnea, high blood pressure, heart disease, and some forms of cancer.

Primarily fat around the middle is quite concerning. Extra body weight causes extra baggage leading to back problems and in-creasing the strain in the joints, and can contribute to or worsen injuries to ankles, knees, hips, and other vulnerable locations of the body.

Being overweight can be both a cause and a consequence of de-pression and low self- esteem.

Popular current diets are nutritionally unhealthy, imbalanced and in sufficient, without being effective over a long term. Over-weight tends to make one self-critical, this constant dissatisfac-tion raises the stress hormone cortisol, which in turn encourages stress-related eating, which in turn, results in further weight gain & becomes a vicious circle.

The accumulation of fat in the belly results in an apple-shaped body type which relates to diabetes and heart disease.

Hatha Yoga, Pranayama, Mindful meditation, Proper Diet Plan and Law of Attraction plays a major role in fat loss.

**Disclaimer: This book is not intended as a substitute for the medical advice of physicians. The reader should regularly consult a physician in matters relating to his/her health and particularly with respect to any symptoms that may require diagnosis or medical attention. Kunjal Kriya and all Yoga and Pranayama must be done in a guidance of a Yoga instructor. The opinion of some dietitians and nutritionist are included as a reference only.**

# Table of Contents

# *Chapter - 1*

## Lose Your Weight Naturally

Special Hatha Yoga Kunjal Kriya enhance the digestive system & increases metabolism which helps in fat loss and weight reduction.

Kunjal Kriya strengthens our digestive system. If the person regularly performs Kunjal Kriya, then the person becomes young for a long time as well as the body remains fit and energetic.

Today I am going to tell you about Kunjal Kriya which proves to be very beneficial especially for the stomach and weight loss.

According to scientific research, it is said that in one Kunjal Kriya a person Loses 300 gram of weight and I lost 5 kg weight in 2 Kunjal Kriya and 10 kg weight after 4 Kunjal Kriya followed by proper diet plan, Good sleep, Yoga & Pranayama, Mindful Meditation and Law of attraction affirmation tools and it is the real fact what had happened to me.

Kunjal Kriya balances Vata, Pitta, and Kapha which is the root cause of all diseases according to ancient ayurvedic system.

Abdominal diseases like indigestion, gas disorder, Acidity, and constipation are eliminated and the stomach remains clean and digestive power increases.

**Below is step by step guide for practicing Kunjal Kriya.**

First of all, keep a jug of little warm clean water with you.
Wash the hands and take care that the nails are cut.
Sit in Kagasana and place your hands on your knees.

Sit in this position and drink 4-5 glasses of warm water continuously according to your capacity. You can also drink water with a Jug.

Now stand up and join your both legs together and lean forward. Place the left hand on the stomach. Insert the index finger and middle fingers of the right hand into the throat and rub the upper or deep part of your tongue.

By doing this water will start coming out. As soon as the water starts coming out keep the fingers out of the mouth.

If the water stops coming out, repeat the same action. If the water does not come out even after moving the fingers, it means that all the water has been removed.

**Things To Keep In Mind Before Practicing Kunjal Kriya**

Keep in mind that in Kunjal Kriya, the water should not be too hot nor too cold and do not add salt to the water.

Keep the body posture correct while doing it. To do this, stand in forwarding bending direction. It removes water easily from inside.

Take a bath 2 hours after performing Kunjal Kriya. Doing Kunjal Kriya before sunrise is more beneficial.

Do not practice it daily, practice it once in a week. If you have an acidity problem then you can practice it 3 days a week.

Do not practice it during mensuration.

Heart, Asthma patient practice it under an experienced yoga teacher. Hernia patients avoid this.

Eat after 1 hour of practicing this Kriya.

**Benefits of Kunjal Kriya**

Direct effects

At the physical level kunjal can aid the maintenance of good health as well as help in the cure of the following diseases: acidity and gas in the stomach; biliousness, nausea, food poisoning and auto-poisoning; indigestion; inflamed oesophageal mucosa, coughs, asthma, bronchitis and respiratory ailments; headaches, (both tension and migraine) and diseases of the nervous system.

At the pranic level, kunjal gives the whole body a flushing, untying knots and unblocking nadis (psychic nerves which conduct prana) so that the whole body feels revived and alive.

On the mental level, kunjal can help with many types of mental diseases and problems, acting as a kind of shock therapy to recharge the brain and mind. It especially helps with depression, lethargy, apathy, tensions, anxiety, neuroses and phobias.

Indirect effects
The indirect effects of kunjal are that it tones up and helps to rebalance the nervous system, thus helping to rejuvenate the whole body. The energy released by the pranic flush helps tone up the circulatory system, the respiratory system, the urino-genital system and the musculoskeletal system. This is because each system of the body depends upon every other system for its correct balance and smooth functioning. When one system, in this case the digestive system, starts to overflow with energy, this energy spills into the other body compartments and gives them a recharge. The mind and body function as one unit; there is no separating line between them. So when the body is recharged, the mind is also recharged. This explains how mental diseases can be cured through physical techniques. This principle can be applied to all yogic techniques and methods which bring positive energy into our lives.

Physical effects
When we do kunjal, what happens? We stimulate the sensory channels of our nervous system, which sends it signal to the brain. This in turn sends a signal down the motor system to make the body vomit: the diaphragm, stomach and glottis contract, causing the water to move in the reverse direction.

There are three processes of the body which totally paralyse the brain and mind for one moment, leaving you in a 'selfless' state, reminiscent of states of meditation. These are orgasm, sneezing and vomiting. If you think about it and reflect upon your own experiences, you will remember that at the moment of experiencing one of these three states, you felt a wave of energy rush through your body and mind which momentarily stopped all thought and action.

When the brain feels this rush of energy it is in a state of extreme stimulation. Many of its circuits are temporarily cut, leaving only the few most necessary circuits in action. This situation is analogous, but much more gentle, subtle and effective than ECT (electric shock therapy) as used in hospitals for the treatment of depressed patients. Energy floods into every nerve of the brain, but in the case of kunjal, not ECT, it is pranic energy which floods through, giving life and rejuvenating every cell. Then when the energy subsides, these circuits start up again in a more harmonious fashion.

The brain then pours out this energy to the rest of the body via the nerves. This extra energy cleans and purifies by stimulating the cells of the waste-disposal system, and then travels on to the organs of the body. As a result there is a direct increase in body efficiency.

The autonomic nervous system is especially important to our understanding of how physical disease is reduced. It is divided into two parts: the parasympathetic system, concerned with relaxed states of mind, and the sympathetic system, concerned with stress and active times. These two systems constantly balance each other.

For example, when we get into a tense situation or state of mind, the sympathetic system becomes predominant, bringing the adrenals into action. Of course, the parasympathetic system still functions as an undertone, maintaining just enough relaxation in the physical body (reflected down from the mind) so that there is no extreme, and the body can function at its peak.

When you do kunjal, the action of the energy flush moving from the stomach on the physical level, and manipura chakra on the psychic level, stimulates the vagus nerve both in its sensory and motor functions. The vagus is sensory to the heart, lungs, bronchi, trachea, pharynx and digestive tract; and motor to the heart, lungs, bronchi and digestive tract. It feeds directly into the hypothalamus of the brain via its parasympathetic fibres. The hypothalamus controls the whole autonomic nervous system. The vagus is responsible for the gag reflex and vomiting.

The extra energy from kunjal spills into both sympathetic and parasympathetic systems, but as the mind is prepared for vomiting, a stressful situation, the sympathetic predominates. The following results occur: Digestive system : decreased peristalsis and increased glucose into the blood from the liver. Lungs: dilation of the bronchi; stops acute asthma. Salivary glands start secreting and therefore are flushed out and cleaned.

Heart beats faster and the blood vessels dilate giving more oxygen to the heart muscle. The lungs are exercised by the action of the diaphragm and abdomen, which helps breathing and pranayama. Mucus secretions from the mouth, sinuses and lower respiratory tract are stimulated, rinsing out these areas. There is temporary blood rush to the brain which increases oxygen and performance.

*Chapter - 2*

## Jal Neti for Sound Sleep: Sound and Adequate Sleep is very much important for Weight Loss

Jal Neti is a technique that was used by yogis to stay disease-free, and most importantly to use the breath well for their yogic practices without any blockages. Just how brushing the teeth is dental hygiene, the practice of Jal Neti is nasal hygiene. This technique uses water to purify and clean the nasal path, right from the nostrils to the throat.

Jal Neti is one of the six-purification procedures or 'Shatkarmas' mentioned in Hatha Yoga Pradeepika.

**What do you need to do Jal Neti**
A Neti pot
A pinch of salt
Lukewarm water
A Neti pot is usually small and has a long spout on one side, which is small enough to be inserted gently into one of the nostrils during the process.

First of all, take a neti pot with nozzle that can be easily inserted into the nostril.
One teaspoon of salt may be added into half litre of lukewarm water.
Now, fill the neti pot with this water.

**How to do Jal Neti**
The simple steps and technique of performing Jal neti are being given below:

First of all sit in Kagasana having 1 foot distance between legs.
Lean forward from the lower back.
Tilt the head to the opposite side of the nostril whichever is more active at the moment.
Insert the nozzle of the pot into the nostril which is active at that moment.
Open your mouth throughout the neti process and try to breathe through it.
Let the water flow in through one nostril and out through the other nostril.
After finishing half of the water of the Neti pot, put it down and clear your nostril.
The same thing should start from other side.
After finishing from both side, do forceful exhalation from both the nostrils in all the directions i.e. left & right, top & bottom.

## Jal neti practice time

The best time to perform Jalneti is either in the morning or evening.
One must do it at home after competing his job or work.
However, it can be done at anytime of the day.
Those who have blocked or nasal congestion, should perform it many times of the day to prevent germs

## Benefits of Jal Neti

Performing Jala Neti daily keeps your nostrils clean by removing dust, mucus, and different kinds of bacteria.

## Relief from Allergy and Sinus

The most significant advantage of Jala neti is that it helps you to cure sinus infection and allergic reactions. Sinus infection is inflammation of the air cavities, which is present in the passages of the nose. As Jalaneti cleans your nostrils, you will get relief from sinus for sure.

### Improve eyesight

Jala neti can improve eyesight. Many of the problems related to eyes like irritation, night-blindness can be reduced effectively. It also helps to sharpen your vision.

### Cure asthma

Jala neti removes the mucus and dust from nostrils. This practice can also help deliver more oxygen to the lungs. Jala neti is a blessing for asthma patients. If you try this technique daily, you will find a noticeable improvement.

### Smooth breathing

Smooth breathing is essential for lung health. Excessive mucus can obstruct the rhythmic breathing process. Jala neti drains out this excessive mucus and also helps to increase our respiratory volumes.

### Prevent hair issues

Increasing pollution and changing lifestyles have adversely affected the health of our hair. Here Jala neti is going to play a vital role in hair health. By performing this technique in the morning can improve your hair condition. It can reduce hair fall and protect the hair from becoming white/gray prematurely.

### Benefits on mind

While performing Jala neti, excessive heat from our body gets removed; therefore, it helps to lower the mental stress. Also, you will get relief from head-related conditions like a headache, migraine, etc. It can reduce anxiety very effectively. If you perform Jala Neti in the early morning, the concentration levels can get better.

### Say bye to cough and cold

Cough and cold are frequent, especially in the winter and rainy season. Both are respiratory infections and the leading causes of increased mucus production and cough. Jala neti takes care of both cold and cough by removing excessive mucus and keeps the respiratory system healthy.

## Hearing Issues

People who are suffering from ear-related issues, especially hearing problems because of sinusitis, Jala neti is boon for them. Jala Neti can cure a significant kind of infections.

## Overcome Insomnia

Because of the excessive usage of smartphones and digital media, insomnia is now common in the young generation. Jala neti is known to improve sleeping disorders.

## Improve sense of smell

Jala neti can improve your sense of smell effectively.

## Save money

Last but not least. Many people have diseases regarding Lungs, Ear, Nose, Throat, Eyes and many more. They are visiting doctors regularly and spend a lot of money to recover from these diseases. Unfortunately, in most cases, medical treatment fails to cure diseases at the root. Jala Neti is a boon for people, especially those who are suffering from Lungs and ENT diseases. Thus, practicing this technique will give more effective results than any medical treatment. So, instead of wasting money on expensive medical treatments, try Jala Neti once to get long-lasting results.

## Point by point benefits to remember:

Daily practice helps maintain the nasal hygiene by removing the dirt and bacteria trapped along with the mucus in the nostrils.
It soothes the sensitive tissues inside the nose, which can assuage a bout of rhinitis or allergies.
It is beneficial in dealing with asthmatic conditions and making

breathing easier.

It reduces tinnitus and middle ear infections.

It helps abate sinusitis or migraine attack.

It can alleviate upper respiratory complaints like sore throats, tonsils, and dry coughs.

It can clear the eye ducts and improve vision.

Clearing of nasal passages helps improve the sense of smell and thereby improves digestion.

It calms the nervous system and the mind. It also helps relieve stress and brings clarity to the mind.

People have experienced a reduction in their anger by practicing Jal Neti regularly.

It helps improve the quality of your meditation.

It helps improve the quality of your sleep.

**Latest clinical research on Jal Neti benefits:**
While theory always sounds wonderful, jala neti has in fact provided tremendous benefits. The following practical study is an interesting example of the attitude towards the practice in a classic "before and after" way. Also, the study concludes with the actual benefits for varying symptoms in terms of actual percentages.

We hope this study helps to put at rest any apprehensions that one may have about the efficacy of neti.

12 month Study into the Effects of Jala Neti
Upon 200 Yoga Students in Western Sydney
By S. Saraswati

Personal Impressions About Neti Before, During, and After First Trial

| Thoughts or Feelings | Before | During | After |
| --- | --- | --- | --- |
| Positive | 28% | 48% | 76% |
| Negative | 48% | 34% | 18% |
| Mixed | 24% | 18% | 6% |

The above table shows the fact that about half the students had negative impressions before first trying Neti. This is to be expected in cultures such as ours. Comments such as the following were abundant:

Yuk, no way!
Thought I might drown or choke
Skeptical that I could do it
Absolute fear
Gross, not socially acceptable
A good party trick – but you're not really serious
Weird and scary
Disgusting
However, during their first trial, more than half the respondents found the experience of water passing through their nose was not that bad. There were many comments such as:

A bit tingly
Quite pleasant
Not as uncomfortable as I'd imagined
Warm and relaxing
Surprisingly easy
Painless and trouble free
It went through easily
No different to swimming.
After the first trial, three quarters of the practitioners found that Neti was good and beneficial.

Afterwards, these were the typical comments:
Not as bad as I had thought
Clean and fresh feeling
Much clearer breathing
Light headed, but pleasantly so
Could really breathe at last
Smelled things I'd never noticed
Incredible relief from congestion
Great, really alive

Like after a good swim in the surf
Frequency Practised
Less often than alternate days 11%
From daily to alternate days 15%
Once daily 60%
2 - 3 times daily 14%
After some time of regular practice, and by the time they were requested to return their questionnaire 5 weeks later, most students had settled into a routine of every day practice. As expected, these students reported a gradual improvement in their nasal problems. Even beyond the initial health benefits, these people will most probably continue to use Neti as a daily ablution and for illness prevention. The 14% using Neti more than once daily were advised to do so by their yoga teacher for specific therapeutic reasons. Such students needed a big boost to overcome chronic nasal problems, and their questionnaire responses indicated drastic initial changes and then a tapering off of the effects. The 15% who did Neti on average between daily and alternate days, found moderate gains, and most admitted to wanting to do it everyday. "I'd like to but I'm a bit slack". The 11% who did Neti less than alternate days, were either dreadfully forgetful, not really interested, or only did it "when I felt a need to, such as being very blocked up". These were the respondents who had ambivalent or mixed impressions about its healing efficacy.

Reported Short and Long Term Benefits

Short Term
Yes 94%
No  6%
Long Term
Yes 92%
No  8%
We defined "short term" as the first 2 weeks, and "long term" as beyond that. Nearly everyone reported some kind of immediate benefit from the use of Neti. The benefits of Neti, whether

they were further improvement in the initial, known problems, or whether they were unexpected benefits, continued to accrue for some months. A tapering off over time is to be expected due to the drop off rate of "great hopes and new regimes". Also, the effects of Neti become subtler over time, and once over their present health crisis, most people are not interested in continuing preventative health maintenance.

Overall Impression of Neti
After 1 – 2 Months Of Practice

Positive thoughts or feelings 97%
Negative thoughts or feelings 0%
Mixed/unsure thoughts or feelings 3%

Pretty well speaks for itself. An abundance of comments like:

Wish I'd discovered it 50 years ago
Essential to daily health care
Great! I'll be a lifelong user of Neti
I love it – I'm hooked!
Thank You. Neti has changed my life. Even more useful than I imagined. An excellent cleansing method.
I can't understand why doctors don't recommend it.
Should be more widely known
Fantastic way of clearing congestion
Simple, painless, beneficial
Safe and effective cleansing ritual
I can't imagine not doing it forever
Easy, gives a sense of well being
Great for clearer thinking, easier breathing.

**Jal Neti Precautions**
The nose should be dried properly after the process.
People with high blood pressure should be careful during this part. If one feels dizzy while drying the nose, then it should be done standing upright.
Take care that you do not leave any water in the nasal passages as

it might cause an infection.

Like any other yogic practice, learn it from an expert practitioner.

Jal Neti goes beyond nasal cleansing and helps in aligning your body, mind, and soul. Hence, it should be practiced daily and not only when one has a nasal blockage or cold.

Leptin is a hormone that is produced in your fat cells. The less leptin you produce, the more your stomach feels empty. The more ghrelin you produce, the more you stimulate hunger while also reducing the number of calories you burn (your metabolism) and increasing the amount of fat you store. In other words, you need to control leptin and ghrelin to successfully lose weight, but sleep deprivation makes that nearly impossible. Research published in the Journal of Clinical Endocrinology and Metabolism found that sleeping less than six hours triggers the area of your brain that increases your need for food while also depressing leptin and stimulating ghrelin.

If that's not enough, the scientists discovered exactly how sleep loss creates an internal battle that makes it nearly impossible to lose weight. When you don't sleep enough, your cortisol levels rise. This is the stress hormone that is frequently associated with fat gain. Cortisol also activates reward centers in your brain that make you want food. At the same time, the loss of sleep causes your body to produce more ghrelin. A combination of high ghrelin and cortisol shut down the areas of your brain that leave you feeling satisfied after a meal, meaning you feel hungry all the time—even if you just ate a big meal.

Imagine two women you know: One is your model of fitness success (who clearly knows how to slim down correctly and has the body to show for it), and the other is what you fear. This friend has her heart in the right place, but no matter how hard she works, she still struggles with the process and doesn't have the body she wants. The troubling part is that when you talk to both, they share a common approach:

They eat meals that focus on lean protein and vegetables.
They exercise at least three times per week, focusing on both weights and cardio.
They know which foods are truly healthy and which they need to limit—and they do.
And yet one friend—the one who continues to struggle—can't maintain her focus. She has trouble controlling her hunger, always craves sweets, and, despite her biggest efforts in the gym, she doesn't seem to achieve the same results as someone else following the same program.

The problem might seem obvious at first. After all, one woman strays from her diet more than the other. And if exercise "isn't working," it probably means she just doesn't really know how to train.

Sleep Controls Your Diet
The debate about the best way to achieve a healthy weight always revolves around eating and movement. If you want to look better, the most common suggestion is "eat less and move more." But it's not that simple, or even accurate. Sometimes you want to eat less and move more, but it seems impossible to do so. And there might be a good reason: Between living your life, working, and exercising, you're forgetting to sleep enough. Or maybe, more importantly, you don't realize that sleep is the key to being rewarded for your diet and fitness efforts. In fact, around 30 percent of adults don't get enough sleep, according to the Centers for Disease Control and Prevention (CDC). And when you consider that the statistic for obesity is nearly identical, it's easy to connect the dots and discover that the connection is not a coincidence.

Not sleeping enough—less than seven hours of sleep per night—can reduce and undo the benefits of dieting, according to research published in the Annals of Internal Medicine. In the study, dieters were put on different sleep schedules. When their bodies received adequate rest, half of the weight they lost was from fat. However, when they cut back on sleep, the amount of fat lost was cut in half —even though they were on the same diet. What's more, they felt significantly hungrier, were less satisfied after meals, and lacked the energy to exercise. Overall, those on a sleep-deprived diet experienced a 55 percent reduction in fat loss compared to their well-rested counterparts.

Poor Sleep Changes Your Fat Cells
Think about the last time you had a bad night of sleep. How did you feel when you woke up? Exhausted. Dazed. Confused. Maybe even a little grumpy? It's not just your brain and body that feel that way—your fat cells do, too. When your body is sleep-deprived, it suffers from "metabolic grogginess." The term was coined by University of Chicago researchers who analyzed what happened after just four days of poor sleep—something that commonly happens during a busy week. One late night at work leads to two late nights at home, and next thing you know, you're in sleep debt.

But it's just four nights, so how bad could it be? You might be able to cope just fine. After all, coffee does wonders. But the hormones that control your fat cells don't feel the same way.

Within just four days of sleep deprivation, your body's ability to properly use insulin (the master storage hormone) becomes completely disrupted. In fact, the University of Chicago researchers found that insulin sensitivity dropped by more than 30 percent.

Here's why that's bad: When your insulin is functioning well, fat cells remove fatty acids and lipids from your bloodstream and prevent storage. When you become more insulin-resistant, fats (lipids) circulate in your blood and pump out more insulin. Eventually, this excess insulin ends up storing fat in all the wrong places, such as tissues like your liver. And this is exactly how you become fat and suffer from diseases like diabetes.

Lack of Rest Makes You Crave Food

Many people believe that hunger is related to willpower and learning to control the call of your stomach, but that's incorrect. Hunger is controlled by two hormones: leptin and ghrelin.

And it gets worse.

Lack of sleep also pushes you in the direction of the foods you know you shouldn't eat. A study published in Nature Communications found that just one night of sleep deprivation was enough to impair activity in your frontal lobe, which controls complex decision-making.

Ever had a conversation like this?

"I really shouldn't have that extra piece of cake… then again, one slice won't really hurt, right?"

Turns out, sleep deprivation is a little like being drunk. You just don't have the mental clarity to make good complex decisions, specifically with regards to the foods you eat—or foods you want to avoid. This isn't helped by the fact that when you're overtired, you also have increased activity in the amygdala, the reward region of your brain. This is why sleep deprivation destroys all diets; think of the amygdala as mind control—it makes you crave high-calorie foods. Normally you might be able to fight off this desire, but because your insular cortex (another portion of your brain) is weakened due to sleep deprivation, you have trouble fighting the urge and are more likely to indulge in all the wrong foods. (Here's how to eat for better sleep.)

And if all that wasn't enough, research published in Psych neuroendocrinology found that sleep deprivation makes you select greater portion sizes of all foods, further increasing the likelihood of weight gain.

The bottom line: Not enough sleep means you're always hungry, reaching for bigger portions, and desiring every type of food that is bad for you—and you don't have the proper brain functioning to tell yourself, "No!"

Sleep Sabotages Gym Time
Unfortunately, the disastrous impact spreads beyond diet and into your workouts. No matter what your fitness goals are, having some muscle on your body is important. Muscle is the enemy of fat—it helps you burn fat and stay young. But sleep (or lack thereof) is the enemy of muscle. Scientists from Brazil found that sleep debt decreases protein synthesis (your body's ability to make muscle), causes muscle loss, and can lead to a higher incidence of injuries.

Just as important, lack of sleep makes it harder for your body to recover from exercise by slowing down the production of growth hormone—your natural source of anti-aging and fat-burning that also facilitates recovery. This happens in two different ways:

Poor sleep means less slow-wave sleep, which is when the most growth hormone is released.
As previously mentioned, a poor night of rest increases the stress hormone cortisol, which slows down the production of growth hormone. That means that the already reduced production of growth hormone due to lack of slow-wave sleep is further reduced by more cortisol in your system. It's a vicious cycle.
If you're someone who doesn't particularly enjoy exercise, not prioritizing sleep is like getting a physical exam with your father-in-law as the investigating physician: It will make something you don't particularly enjoy almost unbearable. When you're suffering from slept debt, everything you do feels more challenging, specifically your workouts.

The Better Health Secret: Prioritize Sleep
The connection between sleep and weight gain is hard to ignore. Research published in the American Journal of Epidemiology found that women who are sleep-deprived are a third more likely

to gain 33 pounds over the next 16 years than those who receive just seven hours of sleep per night. And with all of the connections to obesity, diabetes, high blood pressure, heart failure, and cognitive failure, the need to sleep goes far beyond just looking better and seeing results from your diet and exercise efforts.

While there's no hard number that applies to all people, a good rule of thumb is to receive between seven and nine hours of sleep per night, and to make sure that one poor night of sleep isn't followed up with a few more. It might not seem like much, but it could make all the difference and mean more than any other health decision you make.

In the table following, our criteria were defined as follows:
- Symptoms Mentioned (Total). Each time a symptom or ailment was mentioned on a questionnaire, either as desiring benefit or as an unexpected benefit of some sort, it was recorded. Many respondents had multiple ailments, some known and some unknown.
- Symptoms, No Change. A percentage count of where there was mention of no improvement + where there was no mention of improvement in an ailment where there was initial mention of desire for improvement.
- Symptoms, Improved. A percentage count of where improvement was noticed in an ailment where there was initial mention of desire for improvement.
- Unexpected Benefits. A percentage count of where improvement was noticed in ailments where there was no initial mention of desire for improvement of that ailment.
- Overall Benefits. The sum of Symptoms Improved + Unexpected Benefits as a percentage of Symptoms Mentioned.

| Symptom or Ailment, or Benefit Gained | Symptoms Mentioned (Total Number) | Symptoms No Change % | Symptoms Improved % | Unexpected Benefits % | Overall Benefits % |
|---|---|---|---|---|---|
| Allergies | 8 | 37 | 25 | 38 | 63 |
| Asthma/Bronchitis | 8 | 50 | 50 | 0 | 50 |
| Chronic Mucus & Catarrh | 7 | 42 | 29 | 29 | 58 |
| Colds | 14 | 21 | 29 | 50 | 79 |
| Ear Problems | 12 | 17 | 17 | 67 | 84 |
| Eye Problems | 8 | 0 | 13 | 88 | 100 |
| General Breathing Difficulties | 103 | 1 | 33 | 66 | 99 |
| ssHay fever | 27 | 15 | 70 | 15 | 85 |
| Headaches (incl. Migraine) | 50 | 8 | 6 | 86 | 92 |
| Nasal Blockages | 55 | 14 | 33 | 53 | 86 |
| Poor Smelling Function | 19 | 5 | 11 | 84 | 95 |
| Post Nasal Drip | 8 | 12 | 75 | 13 | 88 |
| Psychological Imbalances, such as: anxiety, low self confidence, general malaise | 17 | 0 | 0 | 100 | 100 |
| Sinusitis | 49 | 16 | 69 | 15 | 84 |
| Improved Sleep | 7 | 0 | 0 | 100 | 100 |
| Reduction in Smoking | 2 | 0 | 0 | 100 | 100 |
| Spiritual/Meditative Benefits | 15 | 13 | 40 | 47 | 87 |

Chapter- 3

## 4 Pranayama Techniques for Weight Loss

According to weight loss statistics, there are 1 billion overweight adults in the world among which 62.9% have reported exercising is a common method to come out of obesity.

The exercising you choose depends on your obesity level, will power & of course your physical condition. The easiest among all exercising methods is to take conscious breathing i.e. pranayama.

Does effective breathing techniques help in weight loss?

Yes, breathing techniques of pranayama can help you with weight loss! But how does this ancient practice of controlling the flow of Prana works on excess weight gained over the body? Modern science has found answers to it in its own way.

How Does Pranayama Help in Weight Loss?
As we know Pranayama is deep and conscious breathing, in which oxygen supply increased to the cellular community of our body. Due to this increase in the oxygen supply, metabolism becomes super active in the body, thus decreases BMI.

A super active metabolism simply means burning a higher number of calories. The higher the metabolic rate is, quickly you'll lose the weight.

Contents
1. Pranayama Reduces BMI

BMI measuring after pranayama

In a control trial study done by Hampton University researchers, they choose 60 overweight students & divide them into 2 groups.

1st group's overweight students had given 40 minutes deep pranayama breathing class 4 times a week for 3 months.
While another group (control group) overweight students did their normal activities.
Result

On following this for 3 months, the below results are seen:

Average BMI in 1st group decreased from 22.8 to 21.5 (5.7% down)
While in the control group student's BMI increased from 22.3 to 22.4.
This study suggests regularizing pranayama practice in our daily routine doesn't let extra fat accumulate on the body.

But did you get surprised where this extra burns by pranayama, even without sweating through a daily vigorous exercise routine?

2. During Pranayama, Excess Weight Flies as CO2
The fat we get from what we eat is converted into carbon dioxide & water as a residue. So if you're not letting these two side products expelling out, it accumulates in the body in the form of triglyceride (excess fat).

A study published on The BMJ 1 says, In deep breathing, an increased supply of oxygen reacts with fat accumulated into triglyceride while keeping fat-free mass intact.

This chemical reaction shows how triglyceride fat burns in oxidation:

$$C_{55}H_{104}O_6 + 78O_2 \rightarrow 55CO_2 + 52H_2O + energy$$

Now on adding Stoichiometry, In order to oxidize 10 kg of fat, you will need to inhale 29 kg of oxygen that further will produce 28 kg of carbon dioxide.

So if your breathing is deep enough, it means you already expelling extra fat out from the body.

Yoga Breathing for Weight Loss
After reading science explained above, you would have understood the breathing techniques of pranayama has great power to flat your round tummy.

If you're a beginner in pranayama, you can always begin with some preparatory techniques & basics before approaching any individual practice.

However, all the pranayama is beneficial for the body in some way, still, we have covered these special breathing techniques that will double the rate of flattening your tummy.

1. Kapalbhati Pranayama
kapalbhati weight loss

Also known as skull shining breath, comprises active shots of exhalation triggered through the abdomen wall. To do kapalbhati pranayama for weight loss, follow the steps below:

Steps:
Sit in a comfortable meditative posture.
Place your hands on your knees, either free or in Gyan mudra.
Close your eyes and take your first breath slowly in.
Now begin exhaling forcefully so that you feel the inward movement of belly on every exhalation.
If you're a beginner, continue this breathing for 2-3 minutes. An advance practitioner can go for more rounds.

Weight Reducing Benefits of Kapalbhati:

To begin with, Pranayama is the deep-breathing exercise that nourishes the brain. Regular practice of pranayama results in a clear mind, and a refreshing soul. There are different types of

Pranayama exercises, and Kapalbhati is one of them. It is the most effective or the famous of them all. Let us give you the basic introduction of Kapalbhati Pranayama; it is a Sanskrit word where Kapal means 'forehead' and Bhati means 'shining', while Pranayama is a breathing technique. Its benefits are visibly strong and long-lasting.

Kapalbhati helps to cleanse the respiratory system, lungs, and also protects you from allergies and other illnesses. If you practice it regularly, then it strengthens your abdominal muscles and diaphragm. Gain a brighter intellect once you get exposed to the power of inner-wisdom. Not only this but this form of Shat-Kriya technique can energize your entire being.

Initiates Weight Loss

The first and foremost change that we witness in the physical appearance is the reduction in weight. It is a myth that breathing cannot reform your outer image because the tricks and techniques of Kaplabhati help to stretch the muscles of the upper body. Get in shape by contracting your stomach and releasing your breath. Also, increase the time you devote to the practice every day.

Mental Health and Emotional Stability

Notice a shift in your behavior by gaining a more mature vision towards your daily obstacles. Every situation becomes a piece of cake when you imbibe a yogic mindset. Consistent breathing exercises cleanse the mind from the clutter and make your perceptions more transparent. The mental health improves after you make a passage through the breathing exercises for some positive thoughts to rest. It gives emotional stability and harmonization in a relaxing environment.

Better Digestive System and Improved Blood Circulation

Improve your blood circulation by opening the blockages to channelize your energy flow. The chakras are known to align themselves, by reducing concentrated pain on the joints, and by opening the seal for natural energy to transfer. The human organs get rid of the toxins and become a better functioning aid that protects the body from any internal damages. This gives a boost to the digestive system with a simultaneous increase in metabolism. The whole process marks better health and wellness of a human.

Stress-Buster

It may sound fake to the public, but believe it or not; Yoga, Pranayama, Meditation does have a strong impact on the human mind. This activity helps people to bid their goodbye's to stress, anxiety, depression, and also decreases the negative emotions of anger, frustration, etc. A quick tip to calm yourself is to sit idle in one place and to deeply breath-in for a few minutes. Kapalbhati Pranayama relaxes the muscles with its alternative inhalation and exhalation methods.

A beauty hack!

Did you know that Kapalbhati Pranayama gives an instant glow with the shining forehead and better blood circulation? It is definitely a beauty hack since our head needs to circulate blood flow to channelize the energy. So, get a nourished skin a revitalized self by focusing on filtering your mind, body, and soul.

Get rejuvenated with this refreshing activity, give life to your soul with Kapalbhati Pranayama. Appreciate and accept the process of life by staying calm and composed with the practices of Yoga. Replenish thy self with positive thoughts and shine-bright from the inside by carrying a delightful aura. Connect with yourself and hence the nature to get rewarded with a beautiful life. are many benefits of kapalbhati which have a simple working mechanism behind all, is active exhalation & passive inhalation.

In normal breath, our inhale is active & exhale is passive. By making active exhalation, kapalbhati works great for belly fat reduction.

Forcefully exhalation of air activates the abdominal muscles, which helps in the removal of excess fat and toning of the abdomen.

Deep inhalation helps in the pouring of a good amount of oxygen into the circulatory system, which enhances metabolism.

Points to remember:
Avoid exposure to the cold water and air-conditioned surroundings right after the practice.
Research has found that practicing Kapal Bhati pranayama helps in the reduction of waist and hips circumferences, which ultimately helps in weight loss.

2. Anulom Vilom Pranayama
Anulom vilom technique of weight loss

This is another helpful weight-reducing breathing exercise. Due to the use of both the nostrils, one after another 'Anulom vilom' is also known as 'alternate breathing'.

To do alternate breathing for weight loss, follow the below-given steps:

Steps:
Straight your spine & sit comfortably on your mat.
Place left hand over your knee, either freely or in some mudra.
Now close right nostril by thumb inhale from the left nostril,
Next, close the left with the index finger and exhale through your right nostril.
This completes the 'Anulom Vilom' Pranayam. Repeat the practice for 3-4 minutes on a regular basis for the better results.

Weight Reducing Benefits of Anulom Vilom:
Fat acquired due to the hormonal imbalance is settled by long inhalation in anulom vilom. Further, it improves metabolism and ultimately activated endocrine glands.
It removes toxins from the blood, which prevents the supply of oxygenated blood to the fat store muscles.

Points to remember:
One should stop if there is a sudden discomfort during the course of performing this breathing.

Pregnant women should go through the necessary precaution before practicing.


3. Bhramari Pranayama
Humming bee breath weight loss
In this breathing, you need to produce a vibration through the throat. That vibration resembles sound of a bee, this is why 'humming bee breath' is another name of this breathing technique.

To do Bhramari pranayama for weight loss, here are the steps:

Steps:
Sit in a cross-legged posture with spine erect & shoulder relax.
Close your ears with the thumbs and simultaneously close your eyes with the ring and middle finger.
Now, slowly inhale and exhale by creating a sound like a bee, whose vibration should experience throughout your body.
You can also go for advance practice of Bhramari pranayama, when comfortable with basic technique.

After 7-8 rounds, unhurriedly remove your fingers and hands down. Feel the sensation of humming vibration running throughout the whole body.

Weight Reducing Benefits of Bhramari:
Bhramari reduces weight by promoting the secretion of serotonin hormone 2, which acts as a stress buster. Because stress is also a common cause of weight gain, bhramari promotes weight loss action.
It helps in overcoming respiratory ailments, which further promotes deep breathing and ultimately assists metabolic activity.
Pin up the Points:

Heart patient is not advised to retain the breath for too long.
Do not put your thumb inside of your ear canal and try not to put pressure on the cartilage (pinna).

4. Bhastrika Pranayama
Bhastrika pranayama, which means 'Breath of fire' is a very powerful exercise that could burn all your excess fat within a few months.

This pranayama breathing involves the forceful inhalation and exhalation at the same pace.

Steps:
Sit in a comfortable posture (sukhasana, padmasana) & relax your shoulder muscles.
Now, inhale deeply and forcibly while bringing your hands up.
Exhale at the same pace respectively & bring hands down to shoulder level. The duration of the inhale and exhale should be the same in this breathing.
Feel the movement of the abdomen and contraction and relaxation of your diaphragm.
See Here: Detailed instructions of bhastrika

Weight Reducing Benefits of Bhastrika:
Forcible nature of bhastrika pranayama promotes the activeness of the muscles at the physical level, which helps in shedding off the stored fat.
It helps in the detoxification process by purifying the blood from various toxins, which hindered the active metabolism.

Points to remember:
Pregnant women should avoid this breathing practice.
People with the condition of high blood pressure should also avoid the practice.
Do You Have Bad Breathing Habits?
Breath symbolizes the 'Prana', which nourishes your body. Improper reception makes the prana (breath) less utilizable for the rest of the body. Such a situation gives rise to various body ailments. Weight gain is one of the results of bad prana or breathing.

Obese people have a tendency of unconscious breath.

It diminishes their metabolic activity and prevents the cell from excreting fully. Results in, the build-up of toxins in the blood and further supports the weight gaining elements in the body.

Unconscious breath or shallow breath not only bring the less amount of oxygen to the cells but also expells the less amount of $CO_2$ from the blood. This condition promotes various issues regarding weight gain.

$$Chapter - 4$$

## Mindful meditation aids in weight loss

Meditation helps you to reduce weight in a very indirect manner. It reduces stress and calms down your mind and eventually helps you leave unhealthy food habbits which are mostly stress induced. People tend to calm themselves by having more food to relieve their stress which in turn increases their weight. Meditation calms down the stress levels, makes one more aware about ones' thoughts, increases mindfulness and hence helps one give away bad food habbits.

Regarding the type of meditation, irrespective of the method used the aim of every type of meditation is to unfocus on reality and move into nothingless to improve concentration and clarity.

Hence whatever be the method you choose you need to follow some basic rules, which are

Sit comfortably with your back straight but not rigid.
Do it in a quiet place preferably at the same time and same place everyday.

Meditation can help with a lot of things. We are body, soul (mind, will and emotions) and spirit. We spend a lot of time on the body and a small amount of time on our soul but the spirit is quite often neglected. We need to find our spiritual slot what ever that looks like for us, meditation, martial arts, yoga, faith just to name a few and pursue that. If our spirit is weak and sick nothing we do for our body and soul will have lasting effects. Happy searching.

The information I post is for advice only and not a diagnosis. Se

I'm certainly no expert but these methods have helped me tremendously in a very short amount of time. Meditation is simply becoming aware of the present moment, the here and now. This is done by really feeling all physical sensations, from the surface you are sitting on to the texture of your clothes. Just observe how they feel, with no judgement or commentary. Awareness is the only goal.Then listen and really hear all sounds around you. Again, listen with no judgement…if judgements or thoughts come up (a sound annoys you or you start to think about your grocery list), observe it and release it, as though you're watching them pass by.Move your awareness internally to your body. Feel the energy buzzing inside of you, the life energy that allows you to take each breath, the lungs taking in air, the belly that moves in and out as you breathe, the heart that beats in your chest. Feel this energy in your body from your toes all the way through your fingertips.Most of us are all too familiar with the concept of mindless eating. It's what we do when we're sitting in front of the television, engrossed in a project on the computer, scrolling through our phones, or driving. Without thinking, or really even noticing that you're chewing and swallowing, you manage to eat an entire bag of chips or several cookies.

Mindful eating basically boils down to just paying more attention—to your hunger, your cravings, your food, and how your body feels before, during, and after you eat.

When you sit down to your next meal, try incorporating some of these simple techniques.

• Assess (and reassess) your hunger. Before you begin eating, ask yourself how hungry you are on a scale of 1 to 10. After several bites, time to ask yourself again. As the meal progresses, switch to assessing how full you are on a scale of 1 to 10. Aim to stop eating when you are moderately full—around a 7—to help avoid overeating.

• Slow down. Eating more slowly allows you to savor each bite as well as to stay alert to satiety levels. It's no surprise then that a recent six-year study of about 60,000 people found that those who shifted from fast to slow eating had a 42 percent lower rate of obesity during the study period than those who continued to eat quickly.

• Stay focused. Anything that distracts you from concentrating on your food—such as the television, checking social media, reading, or even a lively conversation—can lead to mindlessly overeating.

• Key in to cravings. Rather than trying to talk yourself out of a craving, allow yourself to explore it. Instead of trying to ignore it, notice what the craving feels like in your body, ask yourself what's going on that's triggering it, even spend some time looking at and smelling the food you're craving. Take a few deep breaths, then look at it again to see if it still seems as appealing.

• Savor the first few bites. If, even in a mindful state, you decide you really do want to eat whatever it is you're craving, go ahead. Research has shown that much of the enjoyment of a favorite food is in those first few bites. If you take the time to focus on the sensory experience of those initial bites, you may find that your craving is satisfied without overindulging.

4 WAYS MINDFULNESS CAN HELP YOU LOSE WEIGHT:

1. REDUCE STRESS
Stress can lead to overeating. Mindfulness reduces stress. Try mindfulness meditation to enhance your ability to release worry of the past and concern for the future and be present in and grateful for this moment.

2. STOP AND THINK
Mindfulness and mindful eating helps you recognize why you're eating and when you're full. Check in with your body and your emotions before you reach for that midnight snack and during each daily meal. Ask yourself am I really hungry? Am I feeling full

yet?

## 3. BE PRESENT

Mindfulness and mindful eating allows you to slow down and truly enjoy and be present with your meal and the act of eating. Try eating without talking or doing anything else. No phone, no reading, no TV. Takes small bites, really chew and savor your food.

Think about the origin of your meal. The farmers who farmed, the pickers who picked, the packers who packed, the shippers who shipped, the stockers who stocked, the checkers who checked, the cook who cooked. Thinking about your meal from origin to table will add a whole new dimension to being truly present with your food.

## 4. EMOTIONAL ACCEPTANCE

Emotional over-identification (happy or sad) can lead to over-eating. Mindfulness helps us recognize our emotions and process them in a healthy way through meditation and non-judgmental present moment awareness rather than through food. We are not our emotions, we are not our thoughts, and we are not what we eat either.

# *Chapter - 5*

## Avoid sugar and junk food completely

Here are 11 foods to avoid when you're trying to lose weight.

### 1. French Fries and Potato Chips

Whole potatoes are healthy and filling, but french fries and potato chips are not. They are very high in calories, and it's easy to eat way too many of them.

In observational studies, consuming French fries and potato chips has been linked to weight gain.

One study even found that potato chips may contribute to more weight gain per serving than any other food.

What's more, baked, roasted or fried potatoes may contain cancer-causing substances called acrylamides. Therefore, it's best to eat plain, boiled potatoes.

SUMMARY
French fries and potato chips are unhealthy and fattening. On the other hand, whole, boiled potatoes are very healthy and help fill you up.

### 2. Sugary Drinks

Sugar-sweetened beverages, like soda, are one of the unhealthiest foods on the planet.

They are strongly associated with weight gain and can have disastrous health effects when consumed in excess.

Even though sugary drinks contain a lot of calories, your brain doesn't register them like solid food.

Liquid sugar calories don't make you feel full, and you won't eat less food to compensate. Instead, you end up adding these calories on top of your normal intake.

If you are serious about losing weight, consider giving up sugary drinks completely.

SUMMARY
Sugary drinks can negatively affect your weight and general health. If weight loss is your goal, then giving up soda and similar drinks may have a big impact.

3. White Bread
White bread is highly refined and often contains a lot of added sugar.

It is high on the glycemic index and can spike your blood sugar levels.

One study of 9,267 people found that eating two slices (120 grams) of white bread per day was linked to a 40% greater risk of weight gain and obesity.

Fortunately, there are many healthy alternatives to conventional wheat bread. One is Ezekiel bread, which is probably the healthiest bread on the market.

However, keep in mind that all wheat breads do contain gluten. Some other options include oopsie bread, cornbread and almond flour bread.

SUMMARY
White bread is made from very fine flour, and can spike your blood sugar levels and lead to overeating. However, there are many other types of bread you can eat.


4. Candy Bars

Candy bars are extremely unhealthy. They pack a lot of added sugar, added oils and refined flour into a small package.

Candy bars are high in calories and low in nutrients. An average-sized candy bar covered in chocolate can contain around 200–300 calories, and extra-large bars may contain even more.

Unfortunately, you can find candy bars everywhere. They are even strategically placed in stores in order to tempt consumers into buying them impulsively.

If you are craving a snack, eat a piece of fruit or a handful of nuts instead.

SUMMARY
Candy bars consist of unhealthy ingredients like sugar, refined flour and added oils. They are high in calories, but not very filling.

5. Most Fruit Juices with added sugar
Most fruit juices you find at the supermarket have very little in common with whole fruit.

Fruit juices are highly processed and loaded with sugar.

In fact, they can contain just as much sugar and calories as soda, if not more.

Also, fruit juice usually has no fiber and doesn't require chewing.

This means that a glass of orange juice won't have the same effects on fullness as an orange, making it easy to consume large quantities in a short amount of time.

Stay away from fruit juice and eat whole fruit instead.

SUMMARY
Fruit juice is high in calories and added sugar, but usually contains no fiber. It is best to stick to whole fruit.

6. Pastries, Cookies and Cakes
Pastries, cookies and cakes are packed with unhealthy ingredi-

ents like added sugar and refined flour.

They may also contain artificial trans fats, which are very harmful and linked to many diseases.

Pastries, cookies and cakes are not very satisfying, and you will likely become hungry very quickly after eating these high-calorie, low-nutrient foods.

If you're craving something sweet, reach for a piece of dark chocolate instead.

SUMMARY
Pastries, cookies and cakes often contain large amounts of added sugar, refined flour and sometimes trans fat. These foods are high in calories but not very filling.

7. Some Types of Alcohol (Especially Beer)
Alcohol provides more calories than carbs and protein, or about 7 calories per gram.

However, the evidence for alcohol and weight gain is not clear.

Drinking alcohol in moderation seems to be fine and is actually linked to reduced weight gain. Heavy drinking, on the other hand, is associated with increased weight gain.

The type of alcohol also matters. Beer can cause weight gain, but drinking wine in moderation may actually be beneficial.

SUMMARY
If you are trying to lose weight, you may want to consider cutting back on alcohol or skipping it altogether. Wine in small amounts seems to be fine.

8. Ice Cream
Ice cream is incredibly delicious, but very unhealthy. It is high in calories, and most types are loaded with sugar.

A small portion of ice cream is fine every now and then, but the problem is that it's very easy to consume massive amounts in one sitting.

Consider making your own ice cream, using less sugar and healthier ingredients like full-fat yogurt and fruit.

Also, serve yourself a small portion and put the ice cream away so that you won't end up eating too much.

SUMMARY
Store-bought ice cream is high in sugar, and homemade ice cream is a better alternative. Remember to be mindful of portions, as it's very easy to eat too much ice cream.

9. Pizza
Pizza is a very popular fast food. However, commercially made pizzas also happen to be very unhealthy.

They're extremely high in calories and often contain unhealthy ingredients like highly refined flour and processed meat.

If you want to enjoy a slice of pizza, try making one at home using healthier ingredients. Homemade pizza sauce is also healthier, since supermarket varieties can contain lots of sugar.

Another option is to look for a pizza place that makes healthier pizzas.

SUMMARY
Commercial pizzas are often made from highly refined and processed ingredients. A homemade pizza with healthier ingredients is a much better option.

10. High-Calorie Coffee Drinks
Coffee contains several biologically active substances, most importantly caffeine.

These chemicals can boost your metabolism and increase fat burning, at least in the short term.

However, the negative effects of adding unhealthy ingredients like artificial cream and sugar outweigh these positive effects.

High-calorie coffee drinks are actually no better than soda. They're loaded with empty calories that can equal a whole meal.

If you like coffee, it's best to stick to plain, black coffee when trying to lose weight. Adding a little cream or milk is fine too. Just avoid adding sugar, high-calorie creamers and other unhealthy ingredients.

SUMMARY
Plain, black coffee can be very healthy and help you burn fat. However, high-calorie coffee drinks that contain artificial ingredients are very unhealthy and fattening.

## 11. Foods High in Added Sugar

Added sugar is probably the worst thing in the modern diet. Excess amounts have been linked to some of the most serious diseases in the world today.

Foods high in added sugar usually provide tons of empty calories, but are not very filling.

Examples of foods that may contain massive amounts of added sugar include sugary breakfast cereals, granola bars and low-fat, flavored yogurt.

You should be especially careful when selecting "low-fat" or "fat-free" foods, as manufacturers often add lots of sugar to make up for the flavor that's lost when the fat is removed.

SUMMARY
Added sugar is one of the unhealthiest ingredients in the modern diet. Many products, such as low-fat and fat-free foods, seem healthy but are loaded with sugar.

## The Bottom Line

The worst foods for weight loss are highly processed junk foods. These foods are typically loaded with added sugar, refined wheat and/or added fats.

If you're not sure if a food is healthy or unhealthy, read the label. However, watch out for the different names for sugar and misleading health claims.

Also, remember to consider the serving sizes. Some healthy foods, like nuts, dried fruit and cheese, are high in calories, and it can be very easy to eat too much.

If weight loss is on your mind, you would probably want to achieve your desired weight as quickly as possible! It is a fact that losing weight is just not easy but, with some dietary changes and habits, you can speed up the process. Weight loss includes many things including exercising daily, eating healthy snacks, drinking warm water, etc. We are sure that you know almost everything which one should do in order to lose weight easily and faster but, here, in this article, we are sharing a very little-known home remedy that works when you're on a weight loss journey! Want to know what's that? Just read on!

Garlic and honey
Surely, the combo of garlic and honey may not seem very delicious but, it is very beneficial for your health as well as weight loss. It can improve your overall health conditions. Consuming raw garlic on an empty stomach can also aid digestion and detoxification. Both honey and garlic are one of the healthiest ingredients which can be added in any food. The are many health benefits of honey as well as garlic. So, when you combine them together, what benefits you get out of it?
Health benefits of honey and garlic

1. The combination of honey and garlic can lower your blood pressure and bad cholesterol levels in the body.
2. They can be beneficial in fighting with cold and flu.

3. They can improve your digestion and treat many digestion-related diseases.
4. They can boost your immune system.

5. They can detoxify your body by removing the toxins.

6. They can improve your liver's health.

7. They can be used for treating many types of heart diseases as well as diabetes. How to use garlic and honey for weight loss

You can prepare this weight loss remedy by simply putting honey in a glass jar and then, putting freshly peeled garlic cloves in it. Now, close the lid and give the jar a gentle shake to cover the garlic cloves completely in honey. Let the combo sit for a while and then, eat one clove each morning. Store the rest in the glass jar and consume one each day. One more thing that makes this remedy a must-try for you is that it can improve your skin's health and prevent breakouts because both the ingredients are natural blood purifiers.

So, give it a try and let us know how this worked for you! Do share this with your friends or family members who are trying to lose weight! Thank you for reading, stay healthy!

*Chapter - 6*

## 11 Superfoods for Weight Loss

The human body is designed to be alkaline and it functions properly in this state. The optimum pH for our blood and body tissues is about 7.35 to 7.45. This is slightly above the neutral pH level– between a pH of 0, which is completely acidic, and a pH of 14, which is completely alkaline. However, the foods that most of us eat cause our bodies to be in a constant state of acidity. A constant state of acidity can lead to heart disease, a stroke, cancer, skin disorders, auto-immune conditions, allergies and the list goes on. The solution to this problem is an alkaline diet, which will help balance the pH level of the fluids in the body, including blood and urine. Several foods are alkaline in nature and can help properly balance our pH levels to reduce daily ailments and the possibility of certain long-term health risks.

1. Lemons
2. Cucumbers
3. Celery
4. Avocado
5. Spinach
6. Garlic
7. Kale
8. Broccoli
9. Bell Peppers
10. Wheatgrass
11. Cabbage

1. Lemons

Lemons are extremely high in alkaline minerals, such as potassium, and magnesium that have alkalizing effects on the body. The citric acid in them is highly acidic in a natural state, but once consumed, the citric acid gets metabolized and has a wonderful alkaline effect on the body. Lemons are a good source of calcium, iron and vitamins A, C and B-complex, as well as pectin fibre, and carbohydrates. They also contain potent antibacterial, antiviral and immune-boosting powers. Apart from having a cleansing and detoxifying effect on the body, lemons help improve digestion, aid weight loss, support skin health, boost immunity, fight cancer, control high blood pressure, prevent infections and lots more.

2. Cucumbers

Cucumbers are another healthy addition to an alkaline diet. They can quickly neutralize acids and aid digestion. The nutritional profile of cucumbers is very impressive. They are an excellent source of vitamins K, C and different B vitamins. You also get a good amount of copper, amino acids, carbohydrates, soluble and insoluble fibre, potassium, manganese, phosphorus, magnesium, biotin and silica. Plus, cucumbers are low in calories. They also have antioxidant and anti-inflammatory properties. Including cucumbers in your diet can help reduce your risk of cardiovascular disease, improve digestion, lower blood sugar levels and fight different types of cancer including breast, uterine, ovarian and prostate cancers. Being high in water content, they also keep the body hydrated.

3. Celery

Celery is another very alkaline food you should eat! It can neutralize acids and balance the pH level of your body. It is also a great diuretic, meaning it helps get rid of excess fluid in the body. Plus, being very high in water content, it helps hydrate and nourish the cells in your body. Celery also contains vitamins A,

C, K and some B vitamins, as well as calcium, magnesium, phosphorus, folate, potassium and fibre. Plus, it is low in calories, carbohydrates, fat and cholesterol. This simple green stalk helps lower cholesterol, inhibits several cancers, supports the immune system, fights inflammation, supports cardiovascular health, aids weight loss and lots more.

## 4. Avocado

Avocados are one of the foods you should eat every day. They help flush out acidic waste and promote a more alkaline environment in the body. This creamy, green fruit is packed full of nutrients. Avocados contain dietary fibre, folate, potassium, selenium, and a good amount of healthy fat, along with vitamins K, C, B5 and A. They also contain powerful antioxidants, such as alpha-carotene, beta-carotene, lutein, and more. Adding avocados to your diet will help aid weight loss, fight inflammation, improve your heart health, boost cardiovascular health, fight cancer and provide blood sugar benefits.

## 5. Spinach

Spinach, one of the healthiest leafy greens, is highly alkaline in nature. It is very rich in chlorophyll, which acts as an alkalizing agent and brings your body back to the optimal 7.4 range. Spinach is a good source of vitamins A, B2, C, E and K. It is also loaded with minerals that provide the body with amazing alkaline effects, such as manganese, magnesium, iron, potassium, calcium and folate. Plus, it is loaded with dietary fibre, flavonoids and carotenoids. By eating spinach, you can boost muscle strength, fight anemia, improve heart health, prevent premature aging, reduce your risk of cancer and enjoy healthy skin.

## 6. Garlic

A true miracle food, garlic is another alkaline food that encourages overall good health. The main compound in garlic is allicin, which has antibacterial, antiviral, antifungal and antioxidant properties. Also, garlic has nutrients including vitamins B1, B6 and C, as well as manganese, calcium, copper, selenium and many others. Garlic aids detoxification by increasing production of glutathione that helps filter toxins from the digestive system. This alkaline-forming food offers many other health benefits, too. It promotes cardiovascular health, boosts immune health, lowers blood pressure, supports liver functioning, cleanses the liver, reduces inflammation and fights off cancer, to name a few.

7. Kale

Kale is another alkaline food that you should definitely include in your diet. Kale can balance the acid and alkalize the body. This leafy green vegetable is packed with rich vitamins, such as vitamins A, C and K. It also has nutrients like magnesium, calcium, manganese, copper, potassium, iron, phosphorus and protein. Plus, it offers antioxidant benefits. The fibre and sulfur in kale support the body's natural detoxification process, so that your body can get rid of harmful toxins. It can even lower bad cholesterol, reduce your risk of cancer, improve heart health, aid weight loss, boost immunity and lots more.

8. Broccoli

Broccoli is one of the top alkaline cruciferous vegetables that you should include in your diet. The phytochemicals in broccoli help alkalize the body, increase estrogen metabolism and reduce the symptoms of estrogen dominance. This tasty vegetable is also packed with a variety of vitamins, such as C, K and A. It also has fibre, manganese, potassium, iron, folate and protein. Moreover, it has amazing anti-inflammatory and antioxidant properties. Apart from alkalizing and detoxifying the body, broccoli helps fight cancer, improves digestion, boosts the cardiovascular system, improves immunity, supports skin health, boosts metabolism and lots more.

## 9. Bell Peppers

Be it red, green or yellow, bell peppers are highly alkaline in nature. They help transform acidic foods, raising the body's overall alkaline level.Bell peppers also contain vitamins C, A, B6, E and K, along with potassium, manganese, copper, dietary fibre, folate, iron and several flavonoids that provide powerful antioxidant properties. When eaten regularly, bell peppers help boost immunity, lower hypertension, support eyesight, and increase the body's metabolic rate. They also help decrease the risk of cardiovascular disease, Type 2 diabetes, cancer, inflammation and more.

## 10. Wheatgrass

Another highly alkaline food that people are not aware of is wheatgrass. It's a very strong source of alkalinity as well as several nutrients for the body. It is a rich source of chlorophyll, amino acids and vitamins, such as A, B-complex, C, D and E. It also contains magnesium, potassium, iron, zinc, copper, selenium, thiamine and natural enzymes.Wheatgrass helps in the process of detoxification. It also revitalizes your liver and protects it from environmental pollutants. In addition, it boosts energy levels, improves immunity, aids weight loss, regulates blood sugar levels, improves heart health and fights cancer, to name a few.

## 11. Cabbage

Cabbage offers huge health benefits that can not be ignored! Many health benefits are similar to broccoli (they're in the same plant family).

Cabbage is great for weight loss and beautiful skin! I'm sure you've heard of the cabbage diet (not that I would recommend it). There are only 33 calories in a cup of cooked cabbage, and it is low in fat and high in fiber. Cabbage also helps keep skin looking health, toned, blemish-free and glowing; it's rich in antioxidants (including vitamin C and beta-carotene).

Cabbage is high in beta-carotene, vitamin C and fiber. (Vitamin C to reduce toxins which are the main causes of arthritis, gout, and skin diseases.) Also, cabbage may reduce the risk of some forms of cancer including colorectal cancers.

It's cheap and widely available year-round. There are so many varieties of cabbage, too, including Green, Savoy, red, Napa, bok choy, and Brussels Sprouts (tiny cabbages!). It is possible to enjoy eating cabbage pretty much all year round. Although most any cabbage will work for any use, plant breeders have developed many varieties in many colors and textures. Some are sweet, mild, tender as lettuce; others rock hard and good for shredding or slicing crosswise into thick "steaks" for roasting.

Cabbage lasts longer in the fridge than most vegetables. If cabbage is properly stored, it can last from 3 weeks to up to 2 months in your refrigerator. In optimum root cellar conditions, it can even last longer. Store in a hydrator drawer if possible. Do not remove the outer leaves nor wash until ready to use.

It's versatile. I've sliced it into soups and salads, shredded it into coleslaws, stir-fried it with onions and apples, fermented it into sauerkraut, stuffed whole cabbages or individual cabbage leaves, steamed it, boiled it, fried it, roasted it, and grilled it. I've even experimented with cabbage desserts, not always successfully!

# Chapter - 7

## Black Sesame Seeds with Jaggery helps in Lose Belly Fat

From losing weight to anti-ageing, why you should eat more of 'Til ke laddoos'. Weight loss doesn't always involve going on a hunger strike. Eating sesame seed laddoos made with Jaggery can also help you reduce weight easily as they have fat-burning properties that can help in body toning.

Sesame seed laddoos are rich in zinc, which promotes collagen building and thus helps in anti-ageing and skin toning.
Sweets have their own comforting taste during winters. Whether it is biting into a mushy gulab jamun or enjoying the richness of hot gajar ka halwa, winter desserts hold a special place in the culinary world and in our hearts. However, as delectable as the sweets may be, it is important to keep a check on the health metre and make sure that whatever you're intaking in a substantial quantity is not harming your body.

One such dessert that is both tasty and nutritious is Sesame seed laddoos, popularly known as 'Til ke laddoo' which is a winter staple.

Here are a few reasons why you should eat a lot of laddoos this winter as advised by Dietician Apoorva Saini of Santoshiarogyam Diet E Clinic and Dr Sakshi Chopra, bariatric nutritionist, Jaypee Hospital.

* Weight loss doesn't always involve going on a hunger strike. Eating sesame seed laddoos can also help you reduce weight easily as sesame seeds have fat-burning properties that help in body ton-

ing, as per Saini.

* They are rich in zinc, which promotes collagen building and thus helps in anti-ageing and skin toning.

* Sesame is good for post-menopausal women as the phytonutrients in it regulate and balance the hormonal imbalances.

* The high anti-oxidant content helps prevent cancer and boosts immunity by eradicating free radicals from the body.

* The laddoos are super rich in fibre, which improves blood cholesterol and thus helps control hypertension.

* If you're looking for a healthy fat option, these laddoos are it.

* The iron-rich content along with jaggery is beneficial for anaemic women, pregnant women and adolescent girls, according to Dr Chopra.

* Micro-nutrients present in sesame like copper are good for rheumatoid and arthritis. They are also packed with calcium and should be eaten by osteoporosis patients.

Though both the black and white sesame seeds have almost the same composition, the black is a tad bit higher in fibre.

Weight Loss: Sesame seeds also help burn belly fat and lose weight, the healthy way. These seeds come packed with nutrients including protein, fibre, iron, vitamins, and omega-3 fatty acids that help lose weight.

Sesame seeds or til and their nutty flavour have won the hearts of many in the kitchen. These seeds have long been known for their health benefits and medicinal uses, apart from adding flavour and crunch to a dessert, dish or salad. Turns out, sesame seeds also help burn belly fat and lose weight, the healthy way. These seeds come packed with nutrients including protein, fibre, iron, vitamins, and omega-3 fatty acids that help promote healthy skin and hair, flush out toxins, balance the hormones, support cardiovascular health and help cut the bulge. Moreover, they contain two unique compounds, sesamin and sesamolin, powerful lignans that have been proven to lower cholesterol, prevent high blood pressure, and help with weight loss. We tell you what makes sesame seeds the ultimate condiment that could help lose weight and burn belly fat.

Sesame seeds are high in dietary fibre content. It is known that about 100 grams of sesame has over eight grams of fibre present. Fibre plays a crucial role in weight loss as it helps contribute to a healthy digestive system. Moreover, fibre-rich foods help keep your tummy fuller for longer, thereby, preventing you from overeating or binge-eating. Fibre also helps the sugars and fats you eat, to enter the bloodstream at a steady rate, keeping your blood sugar levels in check. As a result, you avoid a sudden crash that can cause you to feel hungry again.

Sesame seeds are low in sodium, which make them helpful in regulating body fluids and prevent fluid retention in the body.

Sesame seeds are rich in lignans that may help burn fat as they cause the body to release more fat-burning liver enzymes. Moreover, lignans are said to inhibit the formation and absorption of cholesterol and decrease fat metabolism.

Sesame seeds or til are known to be an excellent source of protein, which helps increase your metabolic rate and curbs hunger, thereby avoiding excessive calorie consumption and aiding weight loss. In fact, fibre-rich foods can help you lose fat but maintain muscles.

How to use sesame seeds for weight loss and belly fat?

According to the book Healing Foods by DK Publishing, scatter the seeds on steamed vegetables, or add them to salads, stir-fries, baked goods and sandwiches. Include them in your desserts and dishes and enjoy the crunchy goodness that will help you lose weight. Don't forget to eat a balanced diet, engage in exercises and physical activities and lead a healthy lifestyle.

# Chapter-8

## Law of Attraction Affirmation Tools for Weight Loss

The first question is: Can you lose weight by using the Law of Attraction? The answer? Absolutely!

The next question is: Can you lose weight just by thinking "thin thoughts"? The answer? Again absolutely! However…

You knew that "however" would be there didn't you? That's O.K. There's no sense in denying it. Because chances are you didn't believe it when you read it anyway. You may want to believe it but deep down it sounds a little too good to be true.

The good news however, is that it really isn't so far off the mark.

And that is what this article is about. A "real" way to lose weight using the Law of Attraction.

Now I don't want you to be discouraged. Yes, there will be a little action required on your part for the whole weight loss thing to happen, but it will not be nearly as painful as you "think". And the simple reason is because the most important thing we are going to address is the way you "think".

In other words, you are going to learn how to start "thinking thin".

The difference however, is that you are not going to do this in any kind of phony way. You are not going to "think" one way, yet act another and therefore feel as if you are just lying to yourself.

What you are going to do is take at least three or four little physical actions every day combined with "correct thought" that is really going to get that weight loss momentum going.

O.K now I am going to need you to bear with me for a few moments. I am going to list the physical actions you need to take first – then the mental changes – and then we will get to the fun stuff. How to combine them to make them truly effective.

So please do not groan. As you look at each of these physical steps you will realize just how simple they really are. None of them are the least bit expensive, time consuming or difficult. You can easily slip them into you day without even thinking about it.

Physical Steps:
1. Drink More Water. That 's easy enough right? First of all, water is filling. Especially if you drink it right before a meal. It makes you feel fuller and you eat less. Second of all your body needs water. If you normally don't drink enough your body will retain it for future use. Drink more and your body will let it flow through you easily. Plus it constantly cleans out your system. Even your skin will look better when you add more fresh water to your diet.

2. Drink Green Tea – Not only is it naturally filled with Antioxidants, it is also a natural weight loss inducer. You can use caffeinated or decaffeinated. You can drink it hot or cold. And if you are not crazy about its natural flavor, it now comes in a ton of different flavors you can try (beware of sugar factors however). Be sure to drink at least 3 or 4 cups or bottles a day. Again harmless and easy – but very effective and keeps your body running like a well oiled machine.

3. Take vitamin supplements – The more vitamins – the more efficiently your body thrives – the better you feel – the more energy you have – the more calories you burn! Again very simple. Put these vitamins next to your toothbrush to remind you to take them everyday. – Another quickie – takes 10 seconds.

4. Eat Slower. Another solution that takes almost no effort on

your part and in fact makes your meals much more enjoyable. Every time you take a bite of your food, let yourself completely enjoy the experience. Roll it around on your tongue. Enjoy the flavor of it, the texture. Take time to be thankful for the awesome morsel.

Not only does it make your meals so much more enjoyable, but it will also help you to lose weight. The reason being is that it takes about 20 minutes for your brain to register that you're full. If you eat fast, you can continue eating past the point where are in fact, full. If you eat slowly, you have time to realize you are full, and stop on time.

Plus if you slow down, eventually you will simply get tired of eating. If it normally takes you 15 minutes to scoff down an entire meal but now it takes you the same amount of time to eat only half of it – simply out of habit you will be ready to put your fork down at that 15 minute time limit.

5. Always leave a little food on your plate. You may have heard this one before, but believe it or not it actually works! Especially for this particular exercise. Not only are you consuming many less calories over a period of time by doing this every meal, but you are also giving yourself some positive reinforcement as you go along. You will feel much better when you feel as if you didn't just eat your meal "like a pig" but like a real civilized person.

It will also simply reinforce your positive actions towards weight loss each time you push your plate away with a little food left on it. You can say to yourself "See? See how good I am? I didn't have to eat all of it, but I still enjoyed it! – I did good"

6. Eat Smaller Portions More Often. You might have heard of this before as well, but it also works. Like the water example mentioned above, if you continuously replenish your body with what it needs – it will have no reason to keep anything in reserve and will get rid of it. 5 or 6 small meals a day (as opposed to only 2 or 3 huge ones) will give it this constant replenishment.

7. Deep Breathing. Can you lose weight simply by breathing? Again, believe it or not yes! When you learn to breathe properly. If you go online you can find a ton of good deep breathing exercises to try. How will this effect weight loss? That extra oxygen you are gifting your body with is now moving through your bloodstream, slightly increasing your flow, and getting rid of excess waste and fat. All that in a matter of seconds! Again – quick, easy and painless.

8. Exercise. You knew this had to come into it eventually – but this too can be painless and easy. Walking is awesome! Simply incorporate a little more if it into your day. If you take the bus to work simply get off a stop before and walk the rest of the way. Instead of eating at the office cafeteria, go out someplace you can walk back and forth to. Do you have a store 8 blocks away that you normally drive to – or is your kids' school about that far away? Walk instead of driving to get them.(They will enjoy it too – because they will get more one on one time with you as well.) Just do a little something everyday that makes you feel good and positive about yourself. It does not have to be a full hour at the gym (unless you have the option to do that as well. Obviously if you do – go for it!)

9. Eat Better. This is probably the only physical thing that might require a few moments of your time. But even then it will only take you about 15 minutes a week. Put Simply – Plan Your Diet.

It is no mystery why programs like Jenny Craig works so well when it comes to dieting. It is simply because it is so much easier to eat well when you have the proper foods right in front of you for easy access.

So make up your own plan. Pick the healthy foods you do enjoy and build a weeks worth of menus around them. Take chicken or fish for instance. Go online and find 4 or 5 healthy recipes you can make with them. Write down all the ingredients. Buy them at the grocery store all in one shot. This way everything you need is on hand when you need it.

If you would like to take it one step further and spend a little more time each week then take a couple of hours on a Sunday afternoon and prepare your meals in advance. Put them into individual servings and put them in the fridge or freezer. That simple act will ensure you are eating well all week long!

You will totally eliminate the problem of eating junk food or fast food due to lack of time or because you are always on the run.

Also fill the fridge with the fruits you like, with yogurt, with fresh vegetables you can throw in mini zip locks and can take on the run with you.

Do not make a bigger deal out of this than it is. Simply decide to do it once a week and learn to enjoy the process. Watch television or listen to your favorite music while you are doing it. Learn how to truly enjoy the art of cooking.

O.K. So now we have addressed the simple and easy physical steps. Almost all of them take no time at all and are easy to incorporate into your day.

Now we will address the changes you are going to make mentally:

1. Affirmations: You need to come up with a good one that you are going to use at least 3 times a day. Such as: "I am getting thinner and healthier every minute" or "I feel thinner and healthier already" Or even "Wow! I really am getting thinner every day!" Make sure that whichever one you choose makes you feel really good, because like I said, you are going to be saying it at least 3 times a day to yourself every day.

Once as soon as you wake up – at least once during the day and especially once before you to go bed at night.

2. Walk Around "Feeling" thinner:

How would you feel if you were your perfect weight right now?

Would you stand taller? Shoulders back? Would you walk lighter with more bounce or stride more powerfully? Feel your clothes moving easier on your body? How would your face look? Imagine your jaw or cheekbones more defined. As you sit in your chair at work or move around all day continuously feel as if you already are your perfect weight.

When you talk to people, imagine they are looking at this thinner face that is more defined. Suck in your cheeks just a bit when you are working on the computer feeling how your newly defined face feels to you personally. Feel sexy when you are driving. When you are in bed at night imagine lying there with your flat abs and perfectly muscled legs. Move as if you already have those desired body parts. Move them slowly – sensuously – as you shift positions to get comfortable. Truly "feel" absolutely perfect inside and out!

3.Fantasize

Come up with a great fantasy you can think about right before you go to sleep at night.

So what is your fantasy scenario when you have this perfect body? As a man do you imagine the great looking beauty next door catching your muscles gleaming as you work in your backyard unable to look away from you? As a woman do you imagine your dream guy not being able to take his eyes off of you as you stand in your slinky dress at a cocktail party? How about meeting your "movie star" crush in the most unusual circumstances and they are so totally attracted to you. Do you dream of your spouse unable to stop looking at you or unable to keep their hands off of you? Maybe its just your friends looking at you in amazement asking you how you did it, or how you plan on looking for your 20 year reunion. Go for a fantasy that simply makes you feel really good, excited and accomplished.

Now that you have decided on your affirmation, how you "feel" and look physically and your fantasy – we are going to put it all together with the physical actions and make it work.

Here Goes:

You wake up in the morning and say your first affirmation "I am thinner and healthier already!". You take your vitamins and think – "this is keeping me thinner and healthier" You drink your first glass of green tea "this is keeping me thinner and healthier" You get dressed and "feel" thin You walk lighter, stronger, shoulders back "I already feel like I am my perfect weight" You feel your clothes shifting comfortably Lose around you. Your face feels more defined and you already "feel" more attractive You eat your first small meal of the day "this is keeping me thinner and healthier" You drink another glass of water "this is keeping me feeling thinner and healthier" You remember to do a deep breathing exercise "this is making me feel thinner and healthier You get off the bus stop one stop earlier. As you are walking you are thinking "this is making me thinner and healthier – as a matter of fact I feel great!" As you sit at your desk you slightly suck in your cheeks – you sit taller "I really look and feel great!" You walk to lunch "this is making me feel thinner and healthier" You eat very slowly "Every single bite of this meal is absolutely delicious!" You leave some food on your plate "Wow, I am completely full, I enjoyed every bite and by not finishing I am know I am getting thinner and healthier" You have another cup of green tea "this is making me feel thinner and healthier" You restate your affirmation "I am thinner and healthier already!" a few times during the day Continue on your day. Keep saying, thinking and doing these little things that are making you feel so much better. Then as you "gracefully" slip your beautiful healthy body into your bed at night you think about one of your fantasies. How good you look to that dream person. The look of appreciation in their eyes when they look at you, how good and strong and powerful you feel and you know that tomorrow you will look and feel even better!

The next day start again. This time incorporate a few different things into your day. Skip the tea but replace a meal with a health drink. Use the same kinds of words all the time while doing these things like "this is making me thinner and healthier"

So now what thoughts are you going to have when you have just eaten that really fattening meal or had those few drinks? You are going to think "So what? I also drank my water today that is helping me be thinner, took my vitamins today that is making me thinner, took my walk today that is making me be thinner. I used to eat fattening meals all the time – but back then I didn't ever do anything to counteract it. Now I do things all day long to make myself healthy – so a good meal certainly isn't going to hurt me!"

You see there is no reason for negativity, guilt or self loathing here. As long as you are doing constant positive things throughout your day that are helping you feel good, of coarse you are allowed to enjoy the fattening stuff once in awhile.

After all, life isn't supposed to be torture! All it requires is a healthier balance. Stay good most of the time, think positively all of the time and allow yourself to enjoy the heck out of the good stuff when it becomes available.

Now there is only one no-no when it comes to this exercise.

Do not ever get on a scale!

Here is the deal. As you have probably realized when you first start a diet, the weight comes off fairly quickly. After awhile however it will slow down and your body will reach a plateau where it levels out for awhile.

Getting on a scale at this point is like a death sentence!

There is almost no way to ever remain positive when that needle stops moving. That is when all the sabotaging thoughts come in. When you will start saying to yourself "but I did this and this and this. Why bother if it isn't working? It's all a waste of time, etc."

Do not ever give yourself that opportunity to sabotage yourself. As long as you stay away from that scale you will never be aware if and when that plateau period hits and you will continue to lose weight and feel better about yourself every day. Don't worry. You will know when it is working. When your clothes are swimming on you, when the compliments start coming from every direction, when someone takes a picture of you and for the first time you don't want to rip it up. You don't need no stinkin' scale!

And so there it is. How to really lose weight using the Law of Attraction.

Yes, "thinking thin" does absolutely work as long as you combine it with taking little consistent actions that help reinforce it.

Not to mention that if all of your time and thoughts are on what you are wanting to create, there will be no time or room for any of the old doubts to come through.

So go and get your weight loss momentum going! Believe me it is very addicting and has the strangest side effect of making you feel better in other areas of your life as well.

It is amazing how constant positive thoughts can change just about everything.

# *Epilogue:*

Sipping On Hot Water in the Early Morning Really Help You Lose Belly Fat?

It is not a secret that water is essential for our survival. This is not only because it quenches our thirst, but it is necessary for the proper functioning of the body and keeps diseases at bay.

About 70 per cent of our body is made up of water and to keep our system working efficiently, every individual must consume 2-3 liters of water daily.

Hot water for weight loss

Both cold and hot water have their own set of pros and cons. A glass of cold water helps you to cool down after an intense work-out session, while hot water helps to flush out toxins from the body and allows better digestion of food. Besides, it is commonly believed that drinking water (particularly hot water) can help to shed kilos. In this article, we will tell you how true this claim is.

What studies suggest

As per a research, drinking more water can help a person shed kilos. One reason for this might be because water increases feelings of fullness, helps the body to absorb nutrients, and flush out toxic waste.

As per another study published in 2003, drinking hot water could increase the process of weight loss. The study further elaborated that drinking 500 ml of water before mealtime can increase metabolism by 30 per cent.

Hot water and weight loss

Drinking hot or lukewarm water daily in the morning or throughout the day can assist in weight loss process in three ways.

Boosting metabolism: Drinking hot water alters your body temperature. To compensate for the warm temperature of the water, our body lowers down the internal temperature and activates the metabolism.

Breaks down fat: When trying to shed it is crucial to be careful about fat intake. Hot water breaks down fat in the body and mobilises them to molecules, making it easier for your digestive system to burn them.

Curbs appetite: Warm water helps to curb appetite. Gulping down a glass of warm water 30 minutes before having your meal can help to manage your calories intake.

Other benefits of drinking hot water

Improves digestion: Water acts as a lubricating agent that helps to maintain the smooth flow of the digestion process. It even dissolves food particles that our stomach finds hard to digest.

Calm your nervous system: Hot water can also calm your nervous system. When your nervous system is calm you will feel fewer pains and aches. Moreover, it will help you stay calm and composed throughout the day.

Helps relieve constipation: Hot water contracts your intestine, this reduces the clogging in the intestine, making it easier for the bowel to pass.

Flushes out toxins: Drinking water raises a person's body temperature, which can make them sweat. Sweating removes toxins from the pores.


**About the Author:**

Author has many years of experience in running successful weight loss project with various schools, colleges and universities. Worked several years closely with Ancient Yoga Gurus and applied those wisdom in practical and received huge success in weight loss project. Author also did deep research on the topic from various other sources and finally come up with this book on the basis of his genuine work.

## Could You Help?

I'd love to hear your opinion about my book. In the world of book publishing, there are few things more valuable than honest reviews from a wide variety of readers. Your review will help other readers find out whether my book is for them. It will also help me reach more readers by increasing the visibility of my book.

www.ingramcontent.com/pod-product-compliance
Lightning Source LLC
Chambersburg PA
CBHW051228250726
48655CB00006B/2667